I0408514

Copyright © 2018 by Dr. Oliver Pfaff. All Rights Reserved. No part of this book may be reproduced in any manner without the express written consent of the publisher, except in the case of brief excerpts in critical reviews or articles. All inquiries should be addressed to:

cms-pop@hotmail.com

1st edition: Dr. Oliver Pfaff (May 2019).

The MORINGA Compilation,

KDP Edition

Edited by Jessica Cronin, M.A.

www.thereadersblock.com

jesscronin23@gmail.com

ISBN-13: 978-1542942492

(KDP-Assigned)

Dedicated to biodiversity and

all phenomena of life on Earth

Personal Preface

After my book was basically finished for publishing, I entered the search term "moringa" in Amazon books, just for fun, to check... and I was shocked by the overwhelming amount of books about moringa that already existed.

Flicking through some of these books, it became clear to me that most of them have just a few pages and are quite superficial and basically copied from each other, whereas my book compiles years of experience and investigation, as well as the content of more than one hundred scientific research articles on diverse topics about *Moringa oleifera*.

This is why the book you hold in your hands right now truly can be called **THE Moringa Compilation** and why it doesn't need to fear any competition, whatsoever.

1. Moringa oleifera...

Taxonomic classification:

Kingdom: Plantae

Subkingdom: Tracheobionta

Phylum: Spermatophyta

Division: Magnoliophyta

Class: Eudicots

Subclass: Rosids

Order: Brassicales

Family: Moringaceae

Genus: Moringa

Species: *Moringa oleifera...*

...*Moringa oleifera* is the scientific name of an undemanding tree, native to the southern foothills of the Himalayas in northwestern India. It is fast-growing and drought-resistant and, due to its multiple uses, nowadays is grown in most tropical and subtropical regions.

To traditional Ayurveda medicine, it has been known already for thousands of years with a broad spectrum of uses.

Lately, it has celebrated a rise in popularity due to its wide range of beneficial effects and the solutions it offers to imminent global problems. Similar to Noni (*Morinda citrifolia*), *Moringa oleifera* is considered to have an adaptogenic potential, which means that it has a modulating and harmonizing effect on the performance of the organic systems of living organisms, apart from its known nutritive and specific medicinal values. Responsible for this adaptogenic potential is the unique composition of nutrients and special phytocomponents.

Hundreds of scientific studies have been conducted so far, revealing more and more of the surprisingly wide range of uses of the different parts of the plant. The root, the bark, the leaf, the flower, the pods and the seed, everything can be used for specific means.

In many tropical and subtropical countries, as well as in health-conscientious households in Europe, Canada and the US, Moringa has become an integral part of a balanced, healthy alimentation.

In this book, we will have a closer look at this marvelous plant, also called "Miracle Tree," that can bring blessings of health and wellbeing, not only to us, but also to our pets, livestock and agriculture. It also might increase our harvest yield, or even save our honeybees.

To familiarize ourselves with details, we will let the tree reveal its basic secrets itself.

2. Me, *Moringa oleifera,* and My Family

I am sometimes a torn and feathery-looking evergreen tree with an open crown and drooping fragile branches, especially in rather arid areas, whereas in more moist surroundings, I can be even bushy and leafy.

My foliage is feathery with a tripennate organization of my oval leaves which individually measure, depending on climate and soil conditions, 1 to 3 cm in length. The taste of the young shoots is quite spicy, whereas older leaves are less intense and more fibrous.

I have whitish, sometimes also creamy to pink, 7 to 14 mm flowers with five petals that grow on fine, fluffy, rispen-shaped inflorescences, or flower heads. The sepals are linearly lanceolate and bent backward, and the petals are spatulate-shaped and veined. My flowers have a sweet, unique smell, are edible and can be used for teas. They can even serve as pasture for moringa honey. After being pollinated, I grow long, triangularly-shaped pulleys, like green beans. These can grow up to 80 cm long. Therein the seeds form three, artfully-nested rows, in total about 15 to 40 seeds per bean, which can be harvested and dried for oil production or as prime matter for a flocculant to clump particles together for water purification.

Leaves, flowers and beans, all are edible and can enrich many foods in whatever form, with their different flavors and rich, nutritive contents. So, for example, the unripe fruits can be stewed like beans, which then develop an asparagus-like taste, or the cress-like leaves can be used like spinach as a vegetable. Used as seasoning, they also can spice up meals in fresh or dried form, and, like the flowers, the dried leaves serve to prepare a delicious and healthy tea.

As I am able to use nitrogen from the air, I grow quite fast compared to other trees. In the first year, under ideal conditions, I can grow up to 6m in height, flower and already have my first pods. This means that I am quite productive. After three years, I produce around 3000 to 5000 seeds, or, when trimmed for leaf-production and harvested up to 5 times per year, I produce about 15 kg of fresh leaves, equal to 2 to 3 kg of dried leaf powder per year.

My bark is soft, corky and of a light greyish color. Only on older trunks it might be rough and somewhat darker.

My stem might reach a maximum diameter of around 45 cm in old age of up to 40 years.

Depending on environmental factors, I can reach with my uppermost branches to heights of up to 12 meters.

The straight root with which I ground myself, I also use to tap deep water reserves. It tastes a bit like horseradish. This gave me the western name of "Horseradish Tree." But, there are several other names people have baptized me with, such as "Drumstick Tree," "Miracle Tree," "Mother's Best Friend," and "Life-donor," and, due to the common use in some regions as living fence posts, even, "Fencepost Tree."

Here, just for fun, some original native names in original writing: सहजन (Hindi), ワサビノキ (Japanese), ਸੁਹਾਂਜਨਾ (Punjabi), முருங்கை (Tamil), มะรุม (Thai).

I like most the denomination "Miracle Tree," because it describes the awesome effects the composition of the substances in my leaves, flowers, fruit and bark can induce when used as food, feed, extract or medicine.

My ancestors originally lived in the foothills of the Himalayas in northern India and Pakistan. Especially my species, and two relatives of mine, *Moringa peregrina* and *Moringa stenopetala*, have spread to many foreign places all over the globe.

I am just one of about 33 species of the family of the Moringaceae. Most of them are shrubs and trees native to arid tropical and subtropical Africa. Some of my family are said to be close to extinction due to human activity, such as grazing goat herds in the Sahel, and to increasingly dry conditions induced by climate change.

Based on my exceptional contribution to agriculture and medicine, my species, *Moringa oleifera*, is cultivated all over the tropical and subtropical belt around the world. This means that I am already quite known, at least in the regions where I grow.

I reproduce easily, either with cuttings of my branches or by seed. These should be sowed 2 cm deep in planting bags with a sandy humus mix. The seedlings germinate after 10 to 18 days. To accelerate and assure this process, they can be soaked in tepid water for one day before sowing, and the outer shell of my seeds can be peeled off to help me out.

When I am 10 to 30 cm tall, I prefer being planted where I shall develop for the rest of my life, because I don't stand repotting at all.

3. What I Like and What I Dislike

I usually cannot be repotted, due to the sensitivity of my root system. This means that, once I am grounded out of the seedling bag, I have to be kept in place.

I love direct sunlight, and preferably I grow in loose, deep, sandy and slightly clayey and well-drained soil in an arid climate with an average precipitation of 500 to 1000 mm of annual rainfall. The pH of the soil should be neutral or slightly acidic. This is the situation where I originated from in India and Pakistan.

To feel comfortable, I need an average temperature between 25° to 35° Celsius, although I can stand slightly lower and also higher temperatures, if necessary.

Actually, being grown all over the tropical and subtropical belt, I have also adapted to more moist and rich soils, where I grow leafier and denser; in fact, I am quite adaptable.

Some people in colder climates even grow me on the windowsill or in the greenhouse. Of course I grow quite small there, according to the environmental influences and the size of my pot. At the end of the book, you will find some instructions on how to grow me in a pot on a windowsill.

I don't even need fertilizer, because I use nitrogen captured from the air which, in companionship with some bacteria in my roots, I convert into my own growth promoter. This ability and some special components of mine (auxinas and citoquinas) make me grow quite fast. I can grow up to 6 m in the first year and have flowers and pods with seeds, if not pruned.

This is all due to my very high content of zeatin, a potent plant growth hormone (auxin). Compared to most other plants, I have about a thousand times more of it in my system, especially in my young, sprouting leaves and in my seed.

There is just one thing I cannot stand at all which makes me wither away, rot and die quite fast: wet roots in waterlogged soil.

After the tree has presented its biological peculiarities, let's come back to listen to the scientists and researchers and what they have to say about this very special plant.

We will start to discuss its composition first.

4. Phytochemical Composition

There is the saying that, if you eat moringa regularly, you don't have to worry about consuming optimal nutrients. By far the most nutritious plant in the world, it contains more than 90 health-relevant nutrients, in a natural composition that has synergistic effects and, therefore, are optimally bioavailable.

This is the reason why this tree is called by some researchers the most important plant in human history, because it might play a key role in combating famine in countries with high malnutrition rates, such as the Sahel belt, some Arab countries, or Guatemala and Peru in Latin America.

According to the National Ministry of Health, there are no longer nutrient deficiencies in poor households in

Guatemala that have five moringa plants in the backyard and have learned to use them adequately.

These are the reasons why several authors call moringa a superfood. In fact, it contains nearly all essential and non-essential amino acids in considerable amounts. This is why, in Guatemala, malnutrition is vanishing with moringa.

Due to the fact that its leaves contain all the essential nutrients, vitamins and minerals lacking in malnourished people, and based on the fact that it grows especially well in these regions where famine and malnutrition are the most common, it really might be at least a part of the solution to this imminent, alimentary problem.

Let's have a look at the very often praised, high nutrient values of moringa leaves compared to other standard food products:

Moringa has:

Twice as much high-quality protein as soy

7-times as much Vitamin C as oranges

4-times as much Vitamin A as carrots

17-times as much calcium as milk

25-times as much iron as spinach

15-times as much potassium as bananas

7-times as much Vitamin B1 and B2 as yeast

6-times as many polyphenols as red wine

4-times as much folic acid as bovine liver

4-times as much Vitamin E as wheat germ

Twice as much magnesium as brown millet

Twice as much fiber as whole grain wheat products

1.5-times as many essential amino acids as eggs

At least 26 anti-inflammatory agents

At least 46 antioxidants

High proportions of high-quality fatty acids Omega- 3, -6 and -9

The maximum value of chlorophyll ever measured

The marvelous amount of zeatin (a thousand times more than other plants) and salvestrol.....

....

I found this list in an emotive eBook written by Barbara Simonsohn[1] to support the marketing of a Tenerife-based company producing moringa products for human

---

[1] Simonsohn, Barbara. *Moringa, der essbare Wunderbaum.* 2012. E-book. www.moringa-europa.eu

consumption. Similar lists are rumbling around on the internet with basically the same information. They are actually not wrong, as scientific studies have shown, but they have to be interpreted reasonably and should not be used to sell something by creating a wrong picture for the consumer.

First, we have to take into consideration the bioavailability of these substances. We cannot absorb the full amount of the mentioned nutrients, which were measured in a laboratory, by consuming the listed alimentary products or moringa in whatever form. Just a certain percentage of the total amount is absorbed by our system.

Second, we have to look at the serving sizes. Yes, the serving size of 200 grams of steamed carrots has four-times less Vitamin A, but consuming 200 grams of moringa would require swallowing 400 units of 500 milligram capsules, as commonly sold in containers of 60-120 capsules. This means that it takes at least four complete jars of capsules to get the benefit of 4-times more Vitamin A than is found in 200 grams of steamed carrots.

Nobody does this!

Another question is whether the values are taken from dry leaf powder or fresh leaves. The informative sources dealing with the lists of these values usually don't add this important fact, but this leads to certain differences in the available information.

In the end we can state: Yes, the high nutritive values are very important to supply the body with these mentioned nutrients, if consumed regularly and in considerable amounts, as might happen in countries where the plant grows naturally in the backyard. Whereas, for persons that have only the chance to get dried leaf powder in capsules, these nutritive values are not relevant. In this case, other compounds and mechanisms are responsible for the effects, as will be explained later on.

But there is another way to compare the content of moringa leaves. We can compare its green leaves with the green leaves from other plants. Let's take spinach, which for generations was considered the most nutritious and health-promoting side dish, at least after Popeye conquered the cartoon scene: loved by some but detested by most children, it was a must that every conscious parent put on the table for their kids.

100g of fresh leaves of spinach and moringa contain about:

	Spinach leaves		Moringa leaves	
Protein	3g		10g	X
Calcium	100mg		190mg	X
Iron	2.7mg		4mg	X
Fiber	2.2mg	X	2mg	
Vitamin A	9300IU	X	7570IU	
Thiamine / Vit B1	0.08mg		0.26mg	X
Riboflavin / Vit B2	0.2mg		0.7mg	X
Niacin / Vit B3	0.7mg		2.2mg	X
Vitamin B6	0.2mg		1.2mg	X
Vitamin C	28mg		52mg	X
Potassium / K^+	550mg	X	340mg	

Moringa scores far better than the highly-praised spinach in most categories and, therefore, should be favored as a healthy food ingredient, if available.

The only leafy green that can compete nutritionally with moringa is kale, although moringa wins that battle too, due to its higher Vitamin B levels.

The high nutritious values of the plant parts don't matter much in countries where moringa is basically only consumed in capsules of 500 to 1000 mg, as "leaf powder food supplement" or as dried moringa leaf tea.

There is something else, and something much more important, than the nutrients themselves that make it so valuable in either form. These are the plant hormones (phytohormones), plant enzymes (phyto-enzymes) and other phytocomponents that are effective in small amounts, similar to essential vitamins (organic vital nutrient compounds that an organism requires and usually cannot synthesize itself).

Let's go one by one.

PLANT HORMONES are defined as biochemically-active, organic compounds which, as primary messengers, send signal molecules that control and coordinate the growth and development of the plant and also promote immune response. Since they do not always meet all criteria of hormones, they often are denominated as 'growth regulators.' In addition to the true phytohormones, there are numerous other secondary plant ingredients which also exhibit growth-regulating and allover homeostatic effects. There are, for example, some phenolic compounds and steroids that act not only in the plant itself, but also in other organisms. Therefore, they can be considered as being "universal," comparable to the energetic compound of ATP (adenosine-triphosphate) which is the most important molecule of energy transfer for active processes in all living organisms. From bacteria to human beings, it has proven itself to be the most efficient molecule to take over this task, throughout evolution. This universality of some key substances is the explanation for the observed efficacy of plant extracts as phytomedicine and phyto supplements.

VITAMINS are a quite heterogeneous group of substances usually produced by plants, animals or bacteria that have to be part of our diet to make our system work smoothly. Their ingestion is obligatory, because most of them cannot be synthesized by our body itself. This is why they are essential, and a lack of them leads to deficiency symptoms. Everybody, for sure, is familiar with scurvy, caused by the lack of Vitamin C in sailors of the past centuries.

TRACE ELEMENTS, basically atomic elements or ions also known as OLIGOELEMENTS, are, in their function, vitamin-like, because they hold key positions in different processes and, in association with enzymes, are essential for the appropriate function of our metabolism.

ENZYMES are proteins with specific catalytic effects on biochemical, metabolic processes. This means that they induce them and make them happen, whereby they don't participate directly in the reaction they promote and, thus, can repeat this process many times. This is why only small amounts of enzymes are necessary to transform huge amounts of substrates into a product.

Other PHYTOCOMPONENTS, such as a wide range of alkaloids, flavonoids, polyphenols, glycosides, saponins, tannins and terpenoids, which are known to have multiple positive effects contribute to the richness of moringa. Amongst others, we observe anticarcinogenic, antibacterial, antifungal and adaptogenic impacts that are known but not yet investigated and fully understood.

Sometimes it is quite difficult to isolate certain active substances out of a natural mix extracted from plants that consists of hundreds of components. It is mostly the synergy of the mix that is responsible for its effectiveness, while the mere single substances have not much impact or develop side effects.

The hormones, enzymes, vitamins and trace elements, as well as the other phytocomponents, seem to be one of the reasons why extracts and other products, such as tees or supplements, produced from *Moringa oleifera* are so effective. Some of the substances seemingly are universal and unfold their metabolic action in different species, from plants to animals to human beings. These homeostatic and health-promoting effects can be observed in many plants, but usually not as complete as in 'adaptogenic' species.

Moringa oleifera has plenty of all the essential compounds that are important for the plant itself as integral, functional components, but they also serve as health and vitality-inducing substances for many other organisms. Seemingly, we deal with universal key compounds, not yet fully understood and not yet investigated in detail, but empirically recognized as highly effective. And that is what counts in my opinion. Being effective when applied doesn't necessarily need an explanation. What is important is that it helps. The explanation might come later with the progress of science in the field of investigation of phytoremedies.

Nevertheless, several studies have already shown that *Moringa oleifera* contains various phytochemicals like sulfides, flavonoids, saponins, tannins, terpenoids, glucarates, carotenoids, coumarins, monoterpenes, triterpenes, phenolic acids, indoles, isothiocyanates and alkaloids, amongst others, that have antifungal, antibacterial, bio-enhancing, immune-modulating and adaptogenic activity on plants and animals, as well as on human beings. So, the scientific proof for the explanation of its effectiveness is already on the way via substantiating, empirical experience.

Some of these substances worth mentioning are SALVESTROL, ZEATIN and POLYPHENOLS:

Let's start with SALVESTROL, which reacts positively with the Greek Test, showing hereby its cancer-killing effects. (This test checks the reaction of individual cancer cell tissues from patients on 49 chemo drugs and 50 natural, biological substances).

How does Salvestrol destroy cancer cells? The scientific explanation for this anticancer effect is as follows: When Salvestrol encounters cancer cells in the body, it makes itself available to be metabolized by a specific enzyme that commonly is found within the tumor cells, called CYP1B1 (which, by the way, has become recognized as an important cancer marker). The metabolism of this specific enzyme induces the production of toxins that lead to apoptosis, or cancer cell death. Salvestrol, and the metabolic process it induces, affects tumor cells only, while leaving healthy cells untouched. The result is overall tumor decline and a significant slowing of the formation of metastasis. Salvestrol in supplement form has been shown to affect tumor growth in prostate, lung and bladder cancer, as well as melanoma and breast cancer.

Now, let's have a closer look at ZEATIN, which is one of about 200 known plant cytokines. (Cytokines are proteins which regulate the growth and differentiation of cells and modulate immune system response).

According to the technical, scientific description, zeatin does the following:

1.   Promotes callus initiation when combined with auxins, concentration 1 ppm.

2. Promotes fruit set (the formation of fruit after pollination). Zeatin 100 ppm + GA3 500 ppm + NAA 20 ppm sprayed at 10th, 25th, 40th day after blossom.

3.   Retards yellowing for vegetables, 20 ppm, sprayed.

4.   Causes auxiliary stems to grow and flower.

5.   Stimulates seed germination and seedling growth.

This is just a listing of how this hormone can be used in horticulture.

Zeatin seems to play a key role in making minerals, vitamins, amino acids and all the other nutritive elements bioavailable to cells, facilitating their adsorption through the membrane.

Apart from its adaptogenic and antioxidative effects in human beings, it has been shown to put off apoptosis and to induce cell proliferation. This leads to healthier, more hydrated, youthful skin with fewer wrinkles, if applied in skin care.

Zeatin is a helpful anticancer nutrient, as well. Moringa is the best source for this hormone, due to its 1000-fold concentration compared to other plants, as the zeatin analyses from Lowell J. Fuglie[2] show.

So far, zeatin cannot be synthesized industrially, which makes moringa the only

---

[2] Fuglie, L. J. *The miracle tree: Moringa oleifera, natural nutrition for the tropics.* New York: Church World Service, 1999.

viable, natural source of this substance for the agro, health and cosmetic industries, where it mainly finds its application.

Thanks to zeatin, moringa is a natural cell preservative and cell regenerator, which helps to prevent many diseases mainly caused by oxidative stress.

POLYPHENOLS are micronutrients in our diet, and evidence for their role in the prevention of degenerative diseases, such as cancer and cardiovascular disease, is emerging. The health effects of polyphenols depend on the amount consumed and on their bioavailability. "Polyphenols are a real highlight amongst the phyto components because of their broad spectrum of action," states the author Jean-Michel Mérillon in their book *Bioactive Molecules in Food*[3] This statement describes the difficult-to-name, single effects induced by this broad spectrum of substances belonging to the polyphenols. Basically, their range of action covers anti-cancer, anti-oxidant, anti-microbial, anti-viral, immunomodulatory, anti-inflammatory and cardiovascular preventive responses, shown in different scientific studies.

We know already that polyphenols are much stronger free radical scavengers than Vitamins C, E and ß-carotene, which are known for it. They also reduce the aggregation of blood platelets and prevent the oxidation of fats, which explains their cardiovascular protective effects.

---

[3] Merillon, Jean-Michel and Kishan Gopal Ramawat. *Bioactive Molecules in Food.* Springer Nature Switzerland AG, 2019.

Polyphenols are heat stable and some, such as lycopene for example, actually unfold their full effect by heating.

Finally, we can say that moringa has a very high density of nutrients when compared, weight-wise, with most valuable foodstuff. Additionally, it contains a huge amount of phytosubstances that seem to play key roles in the health-promoting, physiological, homeostatic processes of plants, animals and human beings. It also is proven to have antifungal and antibacterial effects. This makes it highly valuable as feed, food, medicine and as a health-enhancing adaptogen.

Another interesting point to discuss is the incredible antioxidant effect of moringa products. To understand this, we have to clarify what free radicals and their opponents are.

Free radicals are oxygen-containing molecules that are dangerously unstable, because they lack an electron in their chemical structure. They are incomplete, which makes them look for a suitable electron to be complete again. Aggressively, based on the laws of chemistry, they remove the electron they need from the nearest intact molecule (for example, molecules of cell membranes, proteins or DNA). This electron robbery process is called oxidation, which can be seen as part of natural, metabolic processes, but, as soon as it exceeds the tolerable limit, it strains the body and causes oxidative stress. This kind of stress is believed to accelerate the aging process and even to be carcinogenic. Antioxidants are substances that offer the electron and, thus, eliminate the free radicals. Moringa supports our body by keeping free radicals at healthy levels.

ORAC, Oxygen Radical Absorbance Capacity, is an in vitro measurement of the ability of a substance to absorb free radicals, used especially in determining the antioxidant effects of foods.

Moringa shows an extremely high antioxidant capacity with ORAC values of up to more than 100,000 Umol/100g, the highest ever measured. The biological relevance of this value is still to be discussed, because it is measured in vitro, but one can assume it translates into effects in biological systems.

According to my own experiences working with *Moringa oleifera,* I can confirm all the above allegations. I can even add very positive experiences with fermented, aqueous, concentrated leaf extract on plants, chickens and pigs, so far. Soon, I will present my findings on this topic on my webpage: www.oliverpfaff.com.

An important point, not to be forgotten, is the fact that basically all studies conducted regarding the toxicity of concentrated extracts have proved safe for animal models, if not given in completely exaggerated dosages several times a day. Simple sugar (glucose $C_6H_{12}O_6$) in such doses also shows strong toxic effects when applied this way. So, this is not a criterion of toxicity.

In conclusion, we can say that, by empiric experience and proven by reasonable studies, *Moringa oleifera* has proven to be a very healthy food, feed and even medicinal plant whose components are non-toxic.

5. Use as Feed and Fodder

In all rural regions in northern India, Pakistan and parts of the Sahel, where moringa is part of the natural flora, and also in areas where it has been introduced over the course of the last centuries or even just recently, it serves as a highly-nutritive forage plant mainly for goats, sheep and cows. The branches and green shoots get cut, and the animals feed on the leaves and the thin branches. In some places, the material gets triturated and mixed with other feed components or, as happens in some other places like Brazil and India, the material is converted into highly nutritive and fibrous pellets.

Leaves, pods, oil extract and seed cake (what remains after extracting the oil from the seed) are the most commonly used parts of the plant for feed or feed additive.

Moringa is considered one of the most nutritional forage feeds, but, also in dried pellet form, it boasts a richness in basic and essential nutrients and fiber content.

Due to the fact that it basically contains all amino acids in considerable amounts, it is commonly added to feed for dogs, cats, fish and even shrimp in the form of dried feed-flour, flakes or pellets. It is a perfect, natural protein source to be added to different feed types for different animals. Each company that produces feed products from moringa, and each farmer using it, has their own standards and, often, secret recipes. There are, for example, some organic shrimp farmers who discovered moringa as a perfect protein source for their breeding.

As it also contains many essential elements, such as magnesium, potassium and calcium, as well as trace elements such as iron, chromium, cobalt, boron and zinc amongst others, its use reduces the need for other feed supplements. Based on this, we can consider moringa a complete feed product.

Just as an example, two studies conducted in Nicaragua showed that supplementing cattle feed with the leaves and green stems of moringa can increase milk production by 43-65% and can increase daily weight gain in cattle by up to 32%. These are really significant effects.

The adaptogenic effect was not yet taken into account in this consideration, but it cannot be dismissed. Most studies suggest a positive effect beyond the mere result achieved by the presence of the known macro and micro feed components. Most studies attribute this additional effect of better allover performance to the fact that a well-fed and balanced individual has a better immune system and better nutrient utilization. This translates into better feed conversion rates, faster growth, less use of medication, less loss, better quality, and thus, in the end, greater profit; and, all this in a natural and ecological way.

The only negative side to it is the high energy consumption if prepared as pellets, flakes or flour. Whereas, when used as green fodder, this issue does not need to be taken into consideration. The drying of the leaf material has to be done as fast as possible to avoid degradation, fermentation and contamination with fungi. This, as well as the pressing of the pellets, is energy-consuming. Of course, all this can be done with clean and renewable energy which makes it more suitable.

Most farmers and pet owners integrating moringa products into their feed report the already mentioned, positive effects, and also shinier fur, less parasites and, above all, lower veterinary costs.

6. Use as Food

Moringa is a great food ingredient that enriches our cuisine, not only with nutritive content, but also with rich flavors. It makes sense to add this superfood to our list of daily consumption, being aware that conventional produce is low in nutritive value due to modern industrial production methods.

Just to point out, according to David Thomas, who compared the actual mineral density of different vegetables and fruit with values from the 1940s, the figures are alarming. The shares of important minerals have since diminished. In some cases, today we find less than half of the initial values of merely sixty years ago. Broccoli, according to this study, lost about 75% of its calcium in five decades. Equally large is the loss of magnesium in carrots, and, in spinach, the iron content decreased on average about 60%. Also, the mineral losses in fruit are alarming: oranges lost around 67% of their iron content and strawberries 55% of their calcium content.

Sadly enough, the same counts for the vital vitamins as well, also ranging below 50% of the values of some decades ago. Based on these findings we can assume that, even eating "healthy," we might suffer from nutritional deficiencies.

The times when the saying "an apple a day keeps the doctor away" was valid are long gone. To ingest the same amount of Vitamin C that was found in one apple forty years ago, we now need to eat between 5 and 20 apples.

In fact, the decline in nutrients within the food supply is a major contributor to the rise in cancer rates worldwide, because not only macronutrients and vitamins are on the decline, but also other components that help us fight infections and cancer. Salvestrol is just one example. Experts estimate that we consume about just a tenth of the Salvestrol quantities in our diet today that we would have consumed 100 years ago.

So, as a proven bioenhancer and with its bouquet of concentrated nutrients, vitamins, minerals and other phyto-compounds, moringa is a great complementary food and supplement, not only for malnourished people, but also for those of us living in plenty.

It can serve as an overall health-promoting product when integrated into our daily diet. The body selects all it needs from this symphony of nutrients.

There are a wide range of recipes with moringa. Basically, in the regions where moringa grows in the yard, it forms an essential part of the daily diet, be it as a steamed, spinach-like vegetable from young leaves or the unripe pods, similar to green beans with an asparagus-like taste. There are endless ways of integrating leaves, pods, seeds and flowers into daily meals. In the places where moringa doesn't grow and only dried leaf powder, seeds and seed oil are available, it basically serves as a spice for salads, meat or soups, or as tea or an enhancing, immune-modulating, adaptogenic supplement.

Moringa seed oil, also known as Ben oil due to its high content of behenic acid, can enrich salads with its mild taste.

The seeds themselves can even make a great snack, especially when roasted with some salt and perhaps some condiment. But they also can add a tasty kick to a salad or other foodstuff.

Following are some rich recipes for a moringa meal with fresh leaves:

Traditional Indian Kitchari (a thoroughly-cooked mix of rice and other ingredients)

Preparation time: +/- 45 min.

Ingredients:

- Rice (parboiled) or daliya (coarsely ground wheat) = 400 g (14 oz)
- Mixed dal (Legumes that have been stripped of their skin, like lentils, peas, and beans, a fundamental ingredient of the Indian kitchen) = 70 g (2.5 oz)
- Moringa leaves = 100 g (3.5 oz) (or other leafy vegetables)
- Potatoes cut in cubes = 75 g (2.6 oz)

- Pumpkin, green papaya, green beans cut (25 g Each) = 75 g (2.6 oz)
- Oil or ghee = 35 g (1.2 oz)
- Sugar or, even better, Jaggery = 30 g (1 oz)
- Spices and condiments = as per choice
- Water = 250 ml (8,45 fl oz)

Preparation:

a. Roast the properly washed and cut vegetables for 2 to 3 minutes (potato, pumpkin, papaya, beans).
b. Pour water and boil the vegetables until slightly soft but still firm.
c. Add the dal and allow it to boil again.

d. Then add the rice, salt, spices and cook it for about 15 to 20 minutes.

e. Lastly, add the leafy vegetables and moringa leaves and cook until all the ingredients soften.

f. Finally, add the sugar or, to make it more authentic, jaggery and mix well before serving.

Moringa Pesto: Great as a dip or sauce.

Preparation time: 10 min

Ingredients:

- 2 cups basil leaves
- 2 cups of fresh, young moringa leaves. The ratio of basil and moringa can be varied according to taste.
- 2 cloves of garlic
- ½ cup olive oil
- ¼ cup pine nuts (kernels)
- ¼ cup grated parmesan
- 3 teaspoons of lemon juice
- 4 teaspoons of moringa powder, according to taste
- Salt and pepper to taste

Preparation:

a. Place all ingredients in a blender and pulse until smooth.
b. Serve right away with pasta, as a spread or dip, or freeze for later!

Moringa Smoothie: A refreshing sip of health

Preparation time: 5 to 10 min

Ingredients:

- A cup of lamb's lettuce
- A cup of spinach leaves
- A cup of moringa leaves
- 1 apple
- 1 frozen banana
- 2 teaspoons of moringa leaf powder
- Juice of 1 lemon
- 500 ml (16.9 oz or one standard bottle) of pure water

-

Preparation:

a. Place all ingredients in a blender and pulse until a creamy liquid has formed. The banana does not necessarily have to be frozen, but this way it gives the smoothie a freshness kick without using ice cubes.

b. Serve in a glass with some fresh fruit (or biscuits).

Roasted Potato Pancakes with Moringa

Ingredients:

- 500g (17.6 oz) of potatoes
- 1 cut onion or other vegetables according to taste
- 2 eggs
- 1 cup of flour
- 6 tablespoons of moringa powder or fresh moringa (leaves and flowers)
- Salt, pepper and other spices according to taste
- Oil

Preparation:

a. Wash and boil potatoes. Then peel and mash.

b. While the potatoes boil, cut the vegetables into small pieces.

c. Mix all the ingredients with the mashed potatoes and place the dough as flat, circular discs in a lightly-oiled baking pan.

d. Bake in the oven until the surface of the discs are slightly crispy.

For serving, you can sprinkle some cheese and fresh moringa leaves on top.

■■■■■■■■■■■■■■■■■■■■■■■■■■■■■■■■■■

In the same way you use the leaves, you also can use the flowers; they just have a slightly different taste.

The pods can be eaten raw and added to salads when they are about 10 cm long and still green. At the size of an asparagus stem, you can use them the same way and steam them as a vegetable, or you can replace green beans with the cooked moringa pods. You will like it. It is very tasty!

As you see in these four completely different recipes and the description of the use of the flowers and pods, moringa is a very versatile ingredient that can be included in whatever meal you cook.

It is great if you have the chance to get fresh leaves. If not, leaf powder is even more versatile and can be added to whatever you prepare. In the western kitchen, it is used very often as a seasoning for salads, soups or healthy shakes.

Another way to integrate moringa's health-promoting effects in your daily routine is as tea made from dried leaves.

In order to not destroy the positive impact of the relatively thermically-unstable phytocomponents, just boil the water, remove it from the stove and steep the dried and triturated leaves for about 5 minutes before straining. Serve hot, preferably after a meal.

You also can keep this infusion in the fridge and can drink it instead of water, or you can add some freshly pressed lemon or orange juice for a rich, refreshing, blended flavor. The same can be prepared from dried flowers.

The oil from the seeds can be used comparably to truffle oil to enrich salads. Just sprinkle it over the salad and mix it up. You can use it cold for whatever food-enriching purpose, but don't use it to fry, because it will lose its beneficial properties and convert into genuine vegetable oil.

Moringa seed oil is one of the most expensive, usually cold-pressed oils available on the market. This is due to its high content in antioxidant and regenerative substances, which are especially valuable for cosmetics. You can oil your skin directly with it or use it as an ingredient in masks and mixtures you prepare on your own.

Using moringa in whatever form you have available adds some health to your alimentation and, thus, helps to enhance your wellbeing because of its nutritive, and especially of its adaptogenic, effects that will unfold with regular consumption. Just as an example: I know several people who have lowered their blood sugar, cholesterol and triglycerides substantially by drinking a cup of moringa tea after meals as their digestive health elixir.

In summary, we can say that moringa products not only offer health-enhancing alimentation to regions with widespread malnutrition, being an unpretentious plant that grows especially where it is needed most, but it also enriches our dishes as a tasty and health-promoting food complement.

It is especially valuable for expectant and breast feeding mothers, for children and adolescents and for older people; basically for all of us!

7. Use as Adaptogen

First of all, we have to clarify what is meant by an adaptogen as the word seems not to be recognized by autocorrect; it wants to change the noun "adaptogen" into the adjective "adaptive."

Nevertheless, the concept of adaptogens already existed in ancient Ayurvedic medicine, where these health-promoting herbal preparations made from special herbs were called "rasayanas."

A Russian pharmacist (Lazarev 1947) coined the term, but it was not clearly defined until it was worked out by Isreal Brekham, PhD in 1968 who stated that:

1. An adaptogen is nontoxic to the recipient.

2. An adaptogen produces a nonspecific response in the body—an increase in the

power of resistance against multiple stressors including physical, chemical, or biological agents.

3. An adaptogen has a normalizing influence on physiology, irrespective of the direction of change from physiological norms caused by the stressor.

In other words, according to Panossian (1999) it is a: "new class of metabolic regulators (of natural origin) which increase the ability of an organism to adapt to environmental factors and to avoid damage from such factors."[4]

In summary, an adaptogen is a substance that increases the body's non-specific resistance and adaptability to physical and mental stress factors while having a

---

[4] Panossian, AG et al. "Effects of heavy physical exercise and adaptogens on nitric oxide content in human saliva." *Phytomedicine* 6.1 (1999): 17-26.

balancing and strengthening effect on the overall physiology without being significantly toxic.

To make it more clear, if my blood pressure is too high, it will decrease, and if it is too low, it will increase to normal levels by using an adaptogen.

According to literature and according to my own empiric and scientific experiences, these regulating effects occur in all relevant physiological systems which lead to an improvement in the overall wellbeing of the person who consumes moringa products regularly. Additionally, we can observe a general boost of the immune system. It seems to act most effectively when drinking a cup of moringa tea daily. For example, not only cholesterol and triglyceride levels hover in the normal range, but also cold and hay fever can be avoided, even while people around are sneezing and coughing. Since I drink my daily cup of tea, my migraines have vanished and the obligatory seasonal colds have disappeared.

When analyzing these effects, we have to be clear that this has nothing to do directly with the high nutritive values of moringa products or even with the pronounced vitamin levels, because this would mean that a high intake is needed to have these results. It rather has to do with the secondary phytocomponents, such as hormones, cytokines, trace elements and enzymes. The composition of those seems to be the secret that causes the adaptogenic effects. Although several of those substances, such as zeatin, amongst others, are already individually detected and scientifically under investigation to show their adaptogenic potential, we have to be aware of the fact that, if we use these substances separately, taken out of the compound, we increase the danger of provoking negative side effects. This would mean that, although effective, these substances lose the claim of being adaptogenic. We can observe this phenomenon basically wherever science has isolated the active compounds of a plant extract to produce "clean" pharmaceuticals. As an example, I just want to mention the digitalis glycosides present in foxglove. A hundred years ago the apothecary, who still was knowledgeable in natural mixtures, prepared a potent heart remedy for heart insufficiency from this plant. If not overdosed, the medicine had no negative side effects. However, the modern pharmaceutical version can, due to the fact that just one glycoside was taken out of the broad compound (which seems to have a regulatory function) of all the other substances in the plant.

So, we can say that functional bioactive compounds, such as hormones, enzymes, phenolic acids, flavonoids, alkaloids and phytosterols, just to name a few, have a synergistic and harmonizing, even orchestral function that enhances the homeostatic health and wellbeing of the consumer. As these compounds act as key hormones and enzymes, only very small amounts are necessary to induce positive effects. This explains why just a cup of moringa tea, a teaspoon of powder, or even just a few milliliters of extract on a daily basis or an interval regimen unfold its adaptogenic effects.

Basically, this bio-enhancing effect is what we expect from the consumption of moringa products, if we don't need moringa to supplement malnutrition.

All different forms of continuous or intermittent consumption of moringa, whether as food, powder, tea or extracts, will likely induce adaptogenic effects. In this way, all of us can benefit from moringa as a pro-homeostatic, adaptogenic agent to balance our metabolic and enzymatic vital processes, and, thus, create health and wellbeing.

8. Use in Form of Extracts

The production of extracts or tinctures from plants, in all times and cultures, has always been a method to concentrate its immanent healing principles.

Most of the enzymatic and antioxidant phyto-elements that have positive effects on different organisms, such as plants, animals and humans, can be found in concentrated form in the various moringa extracts. Many studies have shown their efficacy.

To clarify, an extract is a substance made by extracting a part of natural, raw materials, such as fruits or leaves, usually by using a solvent, such as ethanol or water.

We can triturate and press the leaves or the seeds to get pure extracts. From leaves, the extract is aqueous and from seeds, we have an oily extract. But, we can also triturate or grind the leaves, seeds or bark and mix this raw material with solvents to extract soluble compounds. These liquid extracts can even be pulverized to obtain a solid concentrate.

Depending on the extracting process, the concentration of the different components found in the extract varies a lot. One factor is the solubility of the components in the solvent used. Another factor is the state of the raw material, which can be fresh leaves or seeds or dried prime matter (air dried, microwave dried or oven dried). The finer the particles of the prime material are, the more concentrated and pure is the primary extract, due to the fact that there is more superficial contact between the material and the solvent.

For the extraction method for small scale production of extracts, the traditional maceration in presence of solvent and subsequent filtering is the most common, followed by the Soxhlet Extraction, which can only be used for thermostable substances. As most active phytocomponents from moringa are thermosensitive proteins and organic acids, maceration, or grinding, and pulverization of the fresh or dried plant material and subsequent exposition to the solvent is the most common way to obtain an extract from moringa.

Most scientific studies have been conducted with ethanolic extracts from dried prime matter that were diluted when applied. In this way, the dose-effect relationship and, thus, the most efficient dose can be determined. In very few studies an aqueous extract had been used. And in just one study, that I know of, both extracts had been compared without any significant difference.

The basic problem of the aqueous extract is its relative instability compared to the ethanolic extract, which is preserved by the solvent itself. This is why the ethanolic extract is more common. In the case of fresh, aqueous extracts, the product has to be used immediately after preparation, which limits its use. Investigating this problem myself, I found a viable way to stabilize aqueous extracts using a special organic process, obtaining even an increased potency of the effects. The explanation for this phenomenon is outstanding for the time being, but I am working on it.

The extracts show a wide range of strong adaptogenic and immune-boosting effects in plants and animals, which can be assumed to occur in human beings, as well. Within the normal range of dosage, in all consulted studies, no toxicity developed.

Bio-enhancing effects have been observed not only from leaf extracts but also from extracts from *Moringa oleifera* pods. This kind of enhancement means that medications are more effective when combined with moringa, probably due to its absorption-facilitating response on drugs, vitamins and nutrients through the gastrointestinal membrane, which leads to an improvement of their bioavailability.

One thing is clear: even in high dilution, the extracts are very effective. In a study conducted by myself in pigs for meat production, the use of medication such as antibiotics could be decreased drastically, up to about 60%, which is a considerable gain both economically and for the health of the meat product. Another study done with weaning pigs shows a scientifically insignificant but, for the commercial pig farmer, economically meaningful weight gain of more than 1 kg when compared to the control group over the same period of time. The data clearly indicate that *Moringa oleifera* extract has a positive, growth-promoting effect on animals. I have observed similar results of higher and healthier yield in poultry, as well.

In plants, the use of a fresh extract from moringa leaves applied as foliar spray, produced directly before application, leads to stronger plant growth, better resistance against plagues and, especially, an up to 35% higher yield with even healthier and tastier fruit.

Here are some examples of the increase in crop yield by moringa plant extract sprayed on the leaves in selected crops in Nicaragua, based on an area of 0.705 hectares, or 1.74 acres, (1 hectare = 2.47 acres) using an aqueous juice extract from green leaves diluted 1/36 with water (according to the study by Foidl, Makkar and Becker): Peanut plants developed bigger flowers, better quality nuts and an increase in harvest from 2.954 kg to 3.750 kg. In soybeans, the plants also had larger flowers, a greater biomass and a higher yield of 2.182 instead of 1.591 kg without spray. Also, the corn harvest was considerably higher with 6.045 kg compared to just 4.454 kg without moringa spray). These are just some examples of the highly significant impact moringa extracts can have when applied properly without additional fertilizer. This is an organic means to increase yield and quality.

These results are very convincing to me, and I can confirm comparable results on an empiric level in my own orchard using a biologically-stabilized aqueous extract.

Finalizing this chapter, we can say that moringa consumed as food can be considered a "superfood." Used as fodder, we can call it a "super fodder." If consumed in smaller amounts, it unfolds its effects as a bioenhancer and adaptogen. Using extracts is a good way to promote the positive, beneficial effects moringa can perform on plants, animals and humans. It can be considered a very effective, health-enhancing supplement.

9. Use as Medicine

Disclaimer: The following descriptions and statements are not intended to replace professional diagnoses and/or treatment.

The use of moringa as a medicinal supplement to maintain and promote health and reestablish Ayurvedic "rasayanas" dates back about four millennia. More detailed written testimony can be found in the "Sushruta Samhita" from the 5th Century BC, the foundation of "modern" Ayurvedic medicine. According to the old scriptures, moringa prevents and heals about 300 ailments and illnesses.

The emphasis in ancient medical practices is not based on the cure of diseases, but on their prevention. Holistic health management and precaution should lead to balanced nutrition and selected physical practice, creating the state of health and wellbeing. The well-trained and wise doctors in ancient China and India received their payment only as long as the population of their village was healthy. Of course, people in those days obeyed their instructions to stay in good shape. Why were ancient doctors so good at preventive methods? Because, to keep their privilege and status, they needed to keep people healthy, and this led them to discover and create the system of Ayurveda and traditional Chinese medicine, which both take a preventive approach. Even in Germany, we know from statistics that one euro spent for prophylaxis spares seven euros of medical costs in the long run.

Based on this background, we have to imagine the use of moringa remedies that developed in folk medicine.

The traditional uses of the different plant parts in folk medicine vary slightly from place to place but are consistent in their basic applications.

Moringa is still used widely in ethnomedicine to treat and prevent health problems. Lately, it has been discovered by Western society as an effective adaptogen to prevent and treat stress, lifestyle and age-related diseases, apart from its culinary value of enriching our meals.

All parts of the plant, such as the flowers, green pods, seeds, seed oil, leaves, bark and roots are used in medicine for a range of different medical purposes.

The employment of these plant parts sometimes differs. In the description below, the uses are summed up in general, mostly without considering the different regional applications.

Let's have a look at these traditional uses that must be contemplated apart from the general adaptogenic effects moringa induces when consumed as a food or supplement.

Not all traditional uses can be confirmed scientifically in studies by modern medicine, but most of the uses have a scientific explanation based on the phytocomponents of the different plant parts.

The list is not complete, as there are many regions worldwide where this plant is widely undocumented in its use for medical purposes.

Moringa flowers in traditional medicine:

• The cold-pressed juice of the whole flower improves the quality and flow of breast milk during lactation in humans and animals.

• This juice also has diuretic and antibacterial effects; thus, it is used to treat urinary tract infections.

• The tea from dried or fresh flowers is a potent immune stimulant used to prevent and treat colds and viral diseases, in general.

Moringa pods in traditional medicine:

• Pods, when consumed raw, are said to help eliminate intestinal parasites, such as worms and tapeworms.

• In traditional Ayurvedic medicine, pods are used when liver and spleen afections are detected.

• Another use is for joint pain, which can be treated with warm wraps from mashed pods.

Moringa seeds in traditional medicine:

• Moringa seeds contain high levels of the antibiotic and antifungal agent pterygospermine and have been shown to be effective against a variety of bacterial infections. Traditionally, they are chewed or swallowed whole for intestinal infections and, for skin infections, a paste of mortared seeds is applied.

• Due to their strong anti-inflammatory properties, seeds are also used for treating arthritis, rheumatism and gout.

• Traditionally, they are also used to treat convulsions such as epilepsy.

• Another field of use is sexual disorders.

• The roasted seeds are given to obtain a diuretic effect.

Moringa leaves in traditional medicine:

• The juice of the leaves is commonly used in many Asian and African countries as a drink to prevent and control malnutrition and its consequences, as well as prediabetes and adult-onset diabetes. The leaves have a blood-glucose lowering effect.

• The leaves, as juice or tea, are used traditionally in India to lower high blood pressure and also to treat diverse states of anxiety.

• The tea also has been shown to lower blood sugar, cholesterol and triglycerides, which makes the tea a panacea for most modern lifestyle diseases.

• The leaf tea is also a very good means to overcome indigestion and to treat gastritis and ulcers.

•When mixed with honey and coconut milk, crushed leaves are used to treat diarrhea and dysenteries.

• The juice from leaves, or leaf powder mixed with carrot juice, has diuretic effects and is used to treat edemas.

• In India and the Philippines, a warm envelope of fresh leaves is placed on swollen glands and joints to reduce inflammation, as moringa contains anti-inflammatory compounds.

• Due to its antibacterial effects, the leaf juice is used to clean and disinfect skin lesions and small injuries.

• In India, based on the traditional Ayurveda approach, the leaves are used to treat fever, bronchitis, eye infections, and middle ear inflammations, and, due to the high Vitamin C content, also to treat scurvy.

• The leaves are also administered to treat intestinal parasites such as amoebas, worms and tapeworms.

• The leaves, in addition to the flowers, are a very popular means to stimulate breast milk production in nursing mothers. That's why the tree also is called "Mother's Best Friend."

- To treat headaches and migraines, the leaves are rubbed against the temples.

Moringa roots in traditional medicine:

The roots are considered to be the most effective medicinal plant part of the moringa tree. However, toxic alkaloids are found below the root bark and, therefore, root-based remedies should only be applied by a knowledgeable person.

- The roots are used as a stimulant for the cardiovascular system and, therefore, should not be used in patients with high blood pressure.

- Since ancient times in India, root-based remedies are used to treat constipation, flatulence and abdominal cramps.

- Another field of application is for colds and fever.

• Bark and roots are also used to prepare medicine for neurological diseases, such as epilepsy, nervous weakness and hysteria.

Usually, in traditional medicine and ethnomedicine the plant parts are used in fresh, mostly macerated form often enriched with other ingredients, either to be eaten for internal and systemic treatments or applied as a wrap for external application.

Dried powder is not as common in ethnomedicine as the fresh plant parts, whereas, in modern phytomedicine, this is the common form to use moringa. The reason for that has basically to do with the availability and the required standardization of the treatment.

Different kinds of tinctures have already been applied for millennia. Nowadays, the use of extracts, especially in agriculture and husbandry for bioenhancing and preventive means, is still under investigation or performed empirically by innovative individuals.

Due to all the collected facts, we can say that moringa is not only an adaptogenic plant that fosters the homeostasis of an organism, but that also has a bioenhancing, immune-stimulating effect, apart from the more specific medical uses.

10. Use for Weight Loss

Moringa is amazing, because, as an adaptogen, it can induce contrasting effects depending on the way it is used. As you can build up your body with moringa due to its highly nutritive composition, you also can lose weight, above all fat, with it.

Considering especially the effects of the green leaves, such as the activation of the metabolic and detoxification processes, as well as the blood sugar and cholesterol-lowering response, they can even help to reduce excess body fat and even stubborn abdominal fat, often known as "love handles" or "beer belly." This cleansing effect combined with healthy nutrition and some exercise generally produces great results, not only physically, but also energetically and emotionally.

To take advantage of this induced fat burning process, you need to use moringa in a specific way. Drink it on an empty stomach in the morning and before going to bed, and use fresh leaves for better results. Of course, all ingredients should come from organic production, so as not to add agrochemical toxins instead of the intended cleansing.

Here is the recipe for your personal weight loss program:

Basic ingredients for a fat-burning moringa health cocktail:

> - 1 cup of water
>
> - 1-1½ cups of fresh cut Moringa leaves, preferably the light green shoots (or two full tablespoons of

dried leaf powder, which is less effective)

- Juice of ½ grapefruit or of ½ lemon (or both)

- A small piece of cucumber

- 1 teaspoon of honey

Preparation: Mix the leaves, the cucumber and the honey in the blender at high speed until you get a smooth, greenish liquid. Then add the juices and shake. Serve in a drinking glass.

Consume this juice daily, preferably in the morning before breakfast and perhaps again before going to bed. As it should be consumed on an empty stomach for best results, you also can consume it 1 hour after any meal.

Of course, you can enrich and vary this basic recipe with a variety of ingredients according to your personal taste and experiences.

11. Use as Cosmetics

Moringa, due to the perfect blend of essential oils, hormones and antioxidants from its different plant parts, is highly effective in strengthening skin, hair and nails when applied externally. The natural and highly-concentrated presence of zeatin, especially, makes it an excellent component for many cosmetic products, such as masks, creams, body milks, moisturizers, soaps and shampoos. This is why we find an endless number of skin care products enriched with moringa. But, in many commercially-produced products, the percentage of active ingredients from moringa is very low. This is why it makes sense to prepare your own moringa skin care products for cosmetic means. In this chapter, you will find some effective and successfully tested recipes you can vary, according to your preferences, for your own spa experience.

Thanks to zeatin, moringa regenerates and strengthens the skin, hair and nails and makes them smoother and more elastic than any other active cosmetic ingredient. Creams enriched with significant amounts of zeatin are extremely expensive, particularly because of the scarcity of this substance which, up to now, could not be produced artificially.

The oil is especially famous, apart from being a very good choice to enrich a Caesar salad, for its skin-caring properties. It smooths and moisturizes the skin while activating repairing mechanisms by inducing natural cell growth. Apart from its effects on the skin, it also helps to prevent, or even to reverse, hair loss and structural hair damage.

The oil should be cold-pressed and from organic, raw material, as all your moringa products should be from a verified, organic source. There is a lot of moringa on the market, but some material, mainly from Asia, cannot even be imported to the US or Europe because of its contamination with agrochemicals, particularly with herbicides and pesticides.

In some places, the mashed leaves are used to accelerate the closure of open wounds. For the same treatment, you can also use very fine ground moringa leaf powder. I have seen some of the miraculous effects of this powder, in some cases mixed with talcum powder, on open diabetic feet or severe decubiti (bed sores) in older patients.

As the active compound of moringa is able to perform such great healing effects on serious health issues, it can also have miraculous rejuvenating and moisturizing effects on skin, in general.. For this, you can use fresh leaves, dried leaf powder, or oil.

But there is even another aspect to this: the effect it has on hair and nails. Moringa seems to reduce hair loss, strengthen hair, and give it a light, glossy texture. Fingernails become strong, nearly to the point of being able to be used as a screwdriver. This effect can be observed in both systemic and external application.

Moringa Avocado Nourishing Skin Mask:

Ingredients:

- 1 tablespoon of fine ground moringa powder
- 1 ripe avocado (mashed)
- 1 tablespoon of honey
- 1 teaspoon of moringa oil (if not available, you can use cold-pressed olive oil)
- 1 teaspoon of lemon juice
- 1 tablespoon of cucumber juice or water

Preparation:

a. Mix all ingredients in a bowl to a smooth paste

b. Apply the paste evenly on your face or the area to be treated (exclude eye area)

c. Leave the mixture on for 10 to 20 minutes

d. Rinse off with warm water; don't use soap. You will immediately feel the nourishing, smoothing and refreshing effect.

This mask can also be used for hair treatment to obtain strong, healthy hair with a brilliant glow. Just follow the same recipe, minus the lemon juice.

If you want to have an effective, healthy, exfoliating scrub, just add, according to preference, oat flakes, rough maize flour, salt, or sugar and double the amounts of the ingredients.

African Moringa Blemish Vanishing Mask:

Ingredients:

- ½ ripe banana
- 1 tablespoon of fine ground moringa powder
- 1 tablespoon of liquid honey
- ¼ to ½ teaspoon of tea tree oil
- A pinch of sodium bicarbonate

Preparation:

a. Mix all ingredients in a bowl to a smooth paste
b. Apply the paste evenly on problem spots with acne or blemished skin (exclude eye area)

c. Leave the mixture on for 10 to 20 minutes

d. Rinse off with lukewarm water; don't use soap. You will feel the calming, anti-inflammatory effect right away. Repeat several times for progressive, long-lasting skin improvement.

There are endless more recipes that can enrich and improve your skin and hair, as well as your overall wellbeing. You can combine and vary them according to your preference and create your own personal health and beauty spa experience at home. And you can be sure that, whatever you enrich with moringa, it will always serve your overall health, wellbeing and vitality. You cannot lose, you can only win. We can even say that moringa, with its anti-aging and rejuvenating effects, is like a "fountain of youth."

12. Use as Flocculant for Water Cleaning

A very interesting aspect of the moringa tree is its wide range of applications. Because, apart from the fact that it can be considered a panacea due to the curative effect on more than 300 ailments and illnesses, as stated in Ayurveda medicine, it has the extraordinary ability to cleanse and convert dirty water into potable water. This is very useful and, sometimes, even crucial in the arid regions where it grows and where, frequently, mud and bacteria-contaminated well water is the only source of drinking water.

Already in ancient times, this purifying effect of the fine ground powder of the moringa seed was used to prepare clean water. The seed flour has a flocculant effect (it forms water-insoluble compounds with water-soluble contaminants, particles and bacteria that then sink to the bottom, leaving clear purified water on top) when mixed with contaminated water. After fifteen minutes, a glass of water can already be freed from suspended particles and bacteria that sink to the bottom of the glass. A bigger water jar can be cleansed within one to two hours as follows: The moringa seed flour is diluted in a glass of water which is then mixed with the water in the bigger container. Constant stirring accelerates the cleansing process. About one hour after you stop stirring, the contaminated particles that bind to the moringa powder settle as sediment at the bottom. Between 70 and 90% of the floating, particle contamination in the water, as well as 90% of bacteria, can be eliminated this way. It is a simple and natural method with a surprising effect as A. Hunde was able to show in 1994 in collaboration with the German-Ethiopian Business Association.

Three hundred households in an Ethiopian village took part in this experiment. One hundred and fifty villagers cleaned their drinking water with 1 to 1.5 moringa seeds per liter, whereas the rest of the villagers drank it untreated, as usual. In the moringa group, gastrointestinal illnesses, such as diarrhea, occurred up to 90% less compared to the control group. This translates into an immense gain of health and wellbeing for the villagers. In addition to the flocculant effect, moringa seed powder acts as an antibacterial agent, which explains this outstanding result. Dr. Joseph Mercola, a famous alternative physician, states that moringa seeds work even better for water purification than many of the conventional synthetic materials in use today.

The antibacterial effect of the seed flour is also used to prevent the infection of superficial wounds by applying it as dry powder or as a paste prepared with water or alcohol.

It is a pity that this knowledge isn't more well-known for the wellbeing of the suffering poor, especially in arid regions where pure drinking water is scarce.

13. Other Uses

The general flocculant effect of the seed powder is also used for more specialized purposes, such as extracting heavy metals and other difficult-to-remove toxins from liquids, for example in black water treatment plants or laboratories. A whole series of investigations about this topic have been conducted by Sanches-Martin et al.[5] showing surprising cleansing properties, even for contaminants that are difficult to eliminate.

Even fluoride, a pollutant that is very laborious to extract and that can make people very sick, which is also often controversially discussed due to the fact

---

[5] Sanchez-Martin, J., J. Beltran and C. Solera-Hernandez. "Anionic Surfactants Removal by Natural Coagulant/Flocculant Products." *Industrial & Engineering Chemistry Research* 48.10 (2009): 5085-5092.

that it is added on purpose to drinking water in some areas, is said to be significantly reduced by the application of moringa seed powder.

The uptake of arsenic (a poisonous metalloid often used in industry and in pesticides, herbicides and insecticides) in soft tissues and blood from contaminated food and drinking water, which has become quite a health concern in some regions, could be reduced drastically by adding moringa seed powder to food.

Amalgam removal accompanied by moringa intake helps to prevent mercury poisoning.

The efficacy of chelation therapy (reduction of contaminants in the blood with molecules called chelates that associate with and, thus, 'catch' toxins) can be increased significantly using Moringa simultaneously.

Another very interesting approach is to use the high reduction capacity of moringa leaf extract, which is responsible for eliminating free radicals, to produce nanoparticles for different uses. Some studies have been conducted comparing the yield of silver nanoparticles using various reductive substances. Moringa is very competitive in efficiency as well as in production cost and in ecological terms. The silver nanoparticles are highly bactericidal and promising for antimicrobial means.

Other nanosubstances produced this way are zinc oxide nanoparticles using *Moringa oleifera* extract as an effective chelating agent.

This green biosynthesis method of employing biological plant extracts to create distinct nanoparticles, whereby moringa extract is one of the best choices, is becoming more and more acknowledged due to its several advantages, such as not requiring additional chemicals and being simple, environmentally friendly, inexpensive and reliable.

Based on its high content of glucosinolates, especially in the roots, they are used to prepare a horseradish replacement for the food industry.

The wood of the moringa tree is not very valuable, but it offers the best firewood characteristics (it burns slowly, producing high temperatures) for cooking or producing charcoal.

In many regions where moringa grows, the tree is used as a natural fence or windbreak hedge, hence the name "fencepost tree." It can create a multipurpose enclosure around a courtyard or along fields. It reduces the dehydration and erosion of soil and gives an often required light shade, letting just enough sunlight through.

Its organic composition and fast growth make it a perfect provider of high-yielding biomass for the production of compost that is rich in nutrients (pure humus, for example) and also for the production of methane in biogas plants.

The runoff from these bio-digesters, where gas is produced in a fermentation process promoted by different microorganisms, is the best fertilizer for agriculture, due to its high concentration of bioavailable plant nutrients.

The seeds can be used not only to provide valuable oil for gourmet use, but also as a substrate for biodiesel production. Several studies have been conducted to assess its viability as an alternative truck fuel with regard to production, yield, and machine compatibility in Australia and other places.

The fact that it grows in arid regions where, usually, not many other trees grow makes it an additional carbon dioxide catcher. When planted in considerable amounts in these regions, it helps to reduce greenhouse gases, especially carbon dioxide, that otherwise accumulate in our atmosphere.

The protection of food from microbial or chemical deterioration has traditionally been an important concern in the food industry, which has been solved with chemically-synthesized preservatives, decreasing both microbial spoilage and the oxidative deterioration of food. The trend of consumers demanding organic solutions has led to the investigation of the ability of several plants and their phytochemicals to tackle this issue. A recent study suggested the antimicrobial and protective effects of moringa seeds as a promising candidate.

14. Negative Effects

We also have to look at the possible negative side effects, or even toxic effects, moringa might have or develop over the time of consumption. Without this, the book would be incomplete.

All the parts of the moringa tree have been safely used by many generations as fodder, food and medicine, but, as with everything, the overuse or exclusive use of just one substance or product over an extended period of time can be harmful.

First of all, we have to recognize that the roots of the plant contain some alkaloids and phytochemical compounds that are powerful toxins. Consumed in large enough quantities as food, it can lead to severe or even fatal intoxications. This is why the root, as well as the bark, should not be consumed as food. It is better used as medicine in controlled quantities, due to its high healing potential, or just as a type of horseradish to replace seasoning in small amounts. Concerning the roots, the amount consumed is crucial for its toxicity.

Looking at the other plant parts, we can state that they are completely safe for regular consumption, as generations of people have proved, although there are scientific findings that suggest the contrary. If we look at these studies closely, very easily we find the WHY of these negative results, because, if we do the same studies with any other product, we will have the same result. Imagine continuously eating only carrots, which are healthy within a balanced diet, but might lead to Vitamin A toxicity when consumed excessively or exclusively.

In the following, I will cite the description of an experimental setup of Aminu Ambi et al. from the Department of Pharmacognosy and Drug Development, Ahmadu Bello University in Zaria, Kaduna-Nigeria. This setup shows the absurdity of these kinds of studies and the conclusions drawn from them.

"A total of 24," (by the way, full statistical significance requires 2000 experimentees), "adult albino (Wister stains) rat, Rattus norvegecus, were grouped into (four I, II III and IV each containing six rats). Group I was fed with 25%, group II was fed with 50% and group III was fed with 75% amended diet containing the powdered leaves of *Moringa oleifera* mixed with standard livestock feed (Growermash) for 93 days." This is a lot, if you consider that their life expectancy is only about 2 Years. "Group IV served as the control and was fed with the standard diet alone. At the end of the experiment, the animals were sacrificed and their vital organs were histopathologically examined. The result of the study revealed that some organs of the treated animals had observable microscopical lesions, while the control animals had no observable microscopic lesions in all the organs examined."[6]

Mr. Aminu's conclusion of these findings is as follows: "It could therefore be concluded that, indiscriminate large consumption of the leaves of *M. oleifera* as both food and

---

[6] Aminu A. Ambi et al., "Toxicity Evaluation of Moringa Oleifera Leaves." *IJPRI* vol. 4 (2011): 22-24. Print.

medicine is not safe for a long period of time."

Everyone with common sense will agree that there is an error in the concept, as the aphorism from Philippus Theophrastus Paracelsus, Swiss physician, alchemist, mystic and philosopher (1493–1541) states: "Alle Dinge sind Gift, und nichts ist ohne Gift. Allein die Dosis macht, daß ein Ding kein Gift ist." Freely transcribed into the English language: "all things are poison, and nothing is without poison. Only the dose makes a thing not poisonous."

We have to be aware that information is manipulation in one way or another. We always have to look at the motives and the concepts behind the source of information. Who is the writer? What is their intention?

How objective is their position?... and so on. Because of this, we need to shape our own opinion about things. There is no such thing as an objective truth out there. It is always at least somewhat biased by the author, because they are looking at the world 'their way,' which means through their own goggles, as I do and as you do, too.

Why should the industry promote a product that is able to replace a whole spectrum of vitamin and mineral supplements, which could destroy a very profitable business?

Never stop using your common sense while reading and investigating whatever subject, and use your capacity for deductive logic. In this way, you bring things more into line and get closer to an objective truth. The same counts for the information about moringa.

15. What Moringa Can Do For YOU

As we are part of evolutive nature, and as all nature is intertwined in a perfect and supportive system as science has lately started to perceive it, we must remember that we cannot live without nature, although nature might live well without us human beings. Our health and wellbeing depends on natural resources.

One of these natural resources is the nutritive and healing composition of the plants that we, as heterotrophic organisms, need to consume to live. The biggest part of our diet consists of vegetable products, such as rice, corn, potatoes, plantains and yams. All these have nutritive value for us. Our complex, homeostatic system needs, for its well and balanced function, a certain set of nutritive and regulative substances.

As our modern nutrition is rather poor and limited, being deficient concerning certain factors, moringa is a natural means to complement this lack.

By integrating moringa produce, whether as food, as a supplement, as natural medicine, or even as cosmetics, we help our system to maintain and recreate health by inducing homeostasis. In this sense, moringa is an overall beneficial and life-enhancing gift of nature.

You won't lose; you can only win by enriching your life with moringa.

In the list below, you will find the scientifically proven and empiric effects of moringa in no particular order:

- It boosts your immune system and, thus, reduces infections and even the incidence of cancer

- It makes nutrients more bioavailable

- It increases performance and endurance

- It increases the effectiveness of several drugs, like some antibiotics, for example

- It has anti-diabetic effects and lowers blood glucose levels

- It is one of the best natural sources of antioxidants (ORAC over 100,000)

- It has anti-inflammatory effects

- It reduces cravings and anxiety

- It increases overall energy levels and activates healthy metabolism and metabolic rate

- It helps keep healthy cholesterol levels

- It is cardiovascularly protective

- It improves brain function

- It combats insomnia

- It regulates thyroid function

- It regulates bowel activity and prevents constipation

- It reduces acids in our system and, thus, equilibrates the acid-base balance

- It helps prevent osteoporosis in advanced age or after menopause

- It improves overall performance

- It helps prevent tiredness and even fibromyalgia

- It lowers levels of toxins, such as arsenic and other heavy metals in the tissues

- It has allover adaptogenic effects on homeostasis and wellbeing

- It can cleanse water and reduce germ and suspended particle content, as well as other contaminants

- It reduces malnutrition in children and adults

- It increases milk production, not only in breastfeeding mothers but also in cows and other mammals

- It has very little anti-nutritional factors as concentrated feed for animals

- It helps to balance the hormonal system in women

- It accelerates the healing of wounds and abrasions by inducing the creation of new tissue

- It is a very complete and nutritious food

-With its blend of orthomolecular components and phyto-constituents, it is an ideal supplement

- It is a very concentrated fodder for ruminants

- It serves as one of the most complete vegetal sources of amino acids

- It increases the yield of staple foods, such as fruits and vegetables, without additional fertilizer up to 35% if applied as foliar spray

- It regenerates, smoothens and strengthens skin, hair and nails

- It has antibacterial properties

- It can be used to reduce substrates in chemical processes, for example in the production of nanoparticles

- It can enrich our everyday food consumption with its gourmet taste

- It can serve as windshield hedge to protect erosion and, meanwhile, serve as fodder

- It can serve as quickly regenerating firewood

- It can serve as biomass for biogas production

....

And now, after this incomplete listing, you still ask what this miraculous plant can do for YOU???

In this chapter, I want to give the tree another chance to direct some words to the reader, as I did in the beginning.

16. My Contribution to the World

Some may say that over billions of years of evolution I developed and became an integrative part of the arid ecosystem of my native habitat between the rolling foothills of the Himalayas. Others may say that I am part of the divine creation to serve a sacred purpose. To me, these opinions are not contradictory; they just describe different reflections of the many-sided gem that represents the truth.

I myself feel a part of creation, and I feel so grateful to serve my fellow beings with the divine gifts my evolutionary creator provided me. I am part of a very diverse ecosystem that includes thousands of other species, from the bacteria, fungus, arthropods and worms my roots share the soil with, to the insects that pollinate my flowers or inhabit the cracks in my bark, to the birds that sing their hallelujah while sitting on my branches, or to other plants that I share the four elements with. They all are, in some way, part of my life and of myself, because I need them and they need me to fulfill the duty each one of us is given within our ecologic niche.

In fact, this is why I don't feel as special as you human beings see me. I basically just fulfill the task our creator gave to me within this marvelous, harmonious balance of nature. I need my surroundings and my fellow companions to perform well and to be able to satisfy the needs of others, especially of the ones that live off and benefit from me. That's all I do: I serve others with the compounds of my body parts as an inexhaustible, infinitely re-growing source of feed, food and medicine, as God foresaw. He gave me the ability to perform as I do. I convert sunlight in the presence of water, carbon dioxide and a long list of other substances and elements into my own components. Each cell in my system is performing its individual task to participate in the oeuvre of creation.

Here I am, ready to serve you, too. Seize it for yourself, your wellbeing and health!

17. How to Grow Me

Before saying farewell and wishing you a healthy and successful future, I want to give you some tips on how to keep me, even in temperate climates, in a pot, on a windowsill, or in a greenhouse.

I love a hot, dry and bright place in the sun for best growth, and, please, water me just moderately and avoid waterlogging. As stated at the beginning of the book, I prefer sandy, light soil that drains well. As you also know, I have a taproot; this is why the size of the pot determines my growth. The bigger the pot, the taller and stronger I will grow.

Early and continuous pruning (in your case probably harvesting leaves) makes me grow even faster, greener and bushier.

You can grow me either out of cuttings or seeds. Both ways are viable, but, if grown from seeds, I develop better roots and grow stronger and healthier in the long run.

To prepare cuttings, you just need some already woody branches. Cut them into 30 to 40 cm-long pieces with an aslant, or angled, cut. You can either dunk the cut end into some root growth-inducing hormone solution before sticking the piece straight or slightly inclined up to half of its length into the soil you have prepared for me, or you stick the branch directly after cutting into the soil. I usually don't need a root growth enhancer because of my natural vitality.

If you have seeds for growing me, you just have to soak them in lukewarm water for one night and bury them about 2 to 3 cm deep in the soil of the pot you want to be the home for my roots for the foreseeable future. In this case, the seeds should germinate within 14 to 21 days after planting, if the surrounding temperature is around 25°C. If it is not warm enough, it might take a bit longer. To accelerate my germination, you can carefully peel off the shell around the seed after soaking them in water.

I usually don't need fertilizer as I am an air nitrogen collector. However, I do need other macronutrients and essential minerals from the soil for healthy plant growth. This is why peat, or soil enriched with peat, is not the best choice for me.

Don't forget that I hate being repotted. If it becomes necessary, try not to touch my root ball when doing so.

When my leaves get yellow and fall off, it is not a sign of approaching autumn but of too much water. I don't usually get sick when my basic needs are met.

An environment of less than 15°C makes my growth stagnate, and I wither away over time.

If these basic rules are applied, you should have a lot of fun with a representative of my species, and you will have a true "kitchen-friend" from which you can harvest healthy and tasty food ingredients or energy boosting teas for long evenings... just on your windowsill, as you might have parsley, sage or thyme.

Enjoy me, benefit from me and promise me that you will help raise consciousness for environmental and health matters amongst your fellow men. Please try to make the world, with your thoughts and deeds, step-by-step a better place to live. This is my message to you, because this is the life lesson our creator entrusted to me: to make the life of others better with my natural means. This is my modest duty, just by obeying my Lord, I even hear people say that I am working wonders. That's why they call me "MIRACLE TREE."

18. Outlook and Challenges

Fifteen years ago there was not much information around about this world-improving tree, whereas nowadays, thanks to the information age of internet and social media, there are now about 15,000,000 hits within 50 seconds searching for moringa in Google. Each hit is an article or piece of information where the word moringa appears. This means that there is quite a lot of material accessible to inform oneself, although, there is also much junk and promotion material just to sell moringa products. However, there are many highly valuable, scientific articles proving the nutritive, antioxidant, bio-enhancing, healing, etc. effects of this plant that is based on serious research. In fact, the latest findings only confirm the ancient knowledge of the Indians and Egyptians and put it into a scientific framework which is understandable and accessible for everyone.

The claim, derived from the ancient Ayurveda, that moringa treats and prevents more than 300 ailments seems to get confirmed continuously by modern science. Many facts are known already, but there is still a long way to go to understand the details of the composition, mode of action and effects of this highly valuable tree. Although, thinking pragmatically, we don't need to know the detailed composition nor the mechanism of action to use and apply moringa and integrate it into our daily routine. We just need to acknowledge what is known up to now.

There are many studies forthcoming that deal with its antimicrobial functions as well as its agro-industrial and pharmaceutical potential. These studies will substantiate further its growing use and consumption worldwide.

Our modern society has to look for suitable and viable solutions to many imminent, man-made problems, such as climate change, shrinking farmland, famine, diminishing water reserves, etc., and I am convinced that moringa can be part of a solution to some of these problems.

The challenge is to spread the information about its broad beneficial uses, especially in the regions where it grows naturally, and to instruct people in its care, as happened in Guatemala, to bring forth a positive and advantageous relationship with the tree.

Education helps overcome dependency on others and creates opportunities. This tree is an opportunity from which everybody can benefit, be it on a personal or on a commercial level, be it just to enrich one's dishes, create health, or to improve the efficiency of a chicken farm or the milk production of a dairy enterprise.

The potential is there, just make it happen!

19. Interesting Sources

There have already been conducted around 1000 scientific studies about *Moringa oleifera*, and the number is growing rapidly. There is an endless amount of information available on the internet.

Everybody can inform themselves about new findings using internet tools such as libraries, scientific journals, and specific pages or YouTube channels.

Valuable scientific studies about moringa and health issues can be found, for example, on the internet platform PubMed at the following address:

http://ncbi.nlm.nih.gov/pubmed (Enter the search term "*Moringa oleifera*")

A collection of documents on different moringa topics can also be found at:

http://www.moringanews.org/

Other interesting sources for information might be:

http://www.treesforlife.org/

http://www.tfljournal.org/

http://www.echotech.org/

http://internationalresearch.webnode.com/

https://youtu.be/ra8kT2ugHbA

By searching the internet, you can confirm what you find in this book, and you can even enter much deeper, and more specifically, into the details of different topics concerning this miraculous tree which is enriching the lives of millions already.

20. Final Words

Moringa oleifera is something like the egg-laying-wool-milk-pork of the vegetable kingdom gifted with healing powers. It is always good to have one of this species at home or, at least, some dried leaf powder or oil in one's kitchen pantry.

Everybody using moringa and integrating its products into their daily routine will benefit from this generous, miraculous plant. It will enrich our life with health, energy, youth...

This is why *Moringa oleifera* deserves a special place in our patio, on our windowsill, or in our kitchen cabinet.

Other books from the author

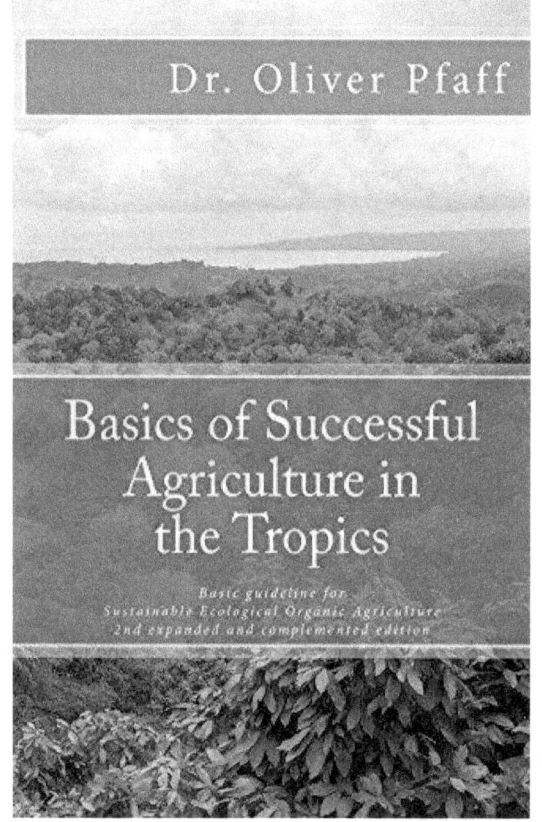

Dr. Oliver Pfaff

Basics of Successful
Agriculture in
the Tropics

*Basic guideline for
Sustainable Ecological Organic Agriculture
2nd expanded and complemented edition*

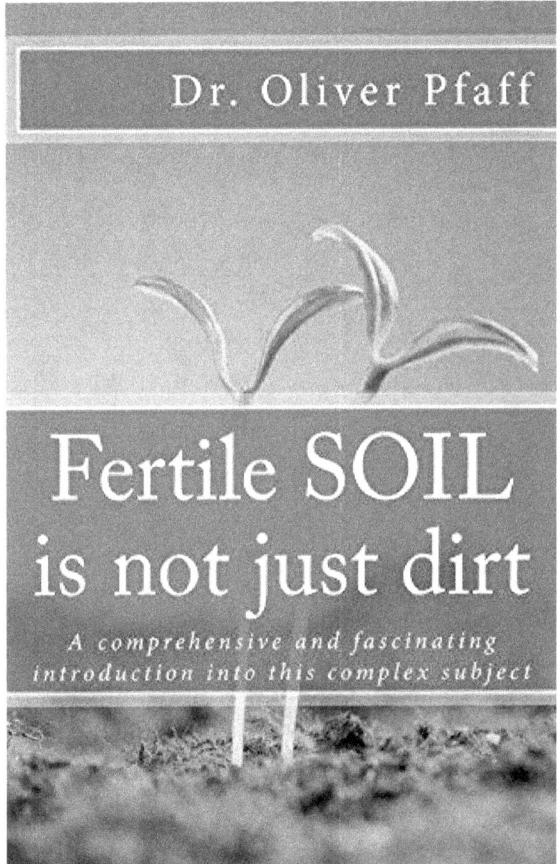

Dr. Oliver Pfaff

Fertile SOIL
is not just dirt

A comprehensive and fascinating
introduction into this complex subject

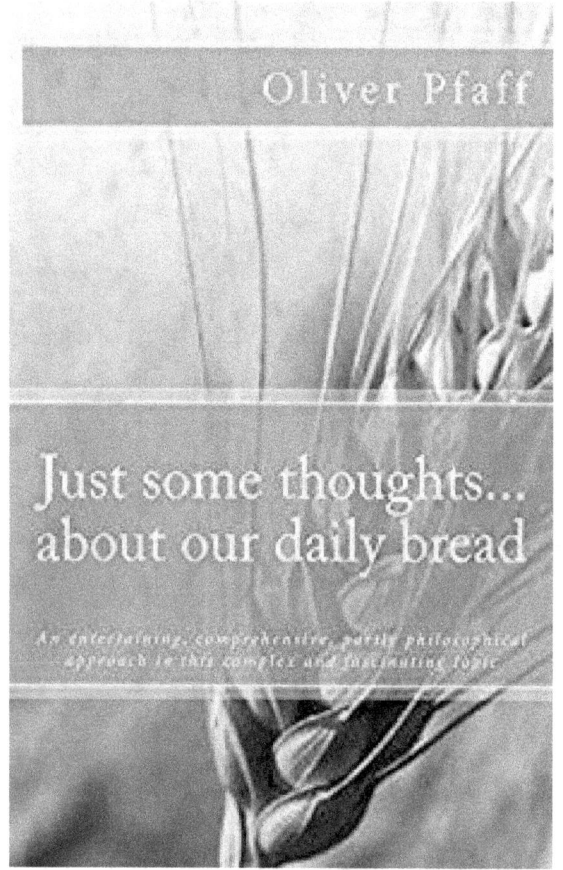

Oliver Pfaff

Just some thoughts...
about our daily bread

An entertaining, comprehensive, partly philosophical
approach to this complex and fascinating topic

www.ingramcontent.com/pod-product-compliance
Lightning Source LLC
Chambersburg PA
CBHW070832310526
45788CB00017B/541